PREGNANCY
PRAYERS

Week by Week Prayers
for You & Your Baby

JAYASRI NAGRALE

with inspiration & guidance from the Archangels

A small note from the Author:

Dear Reader,

Thank you for purchasing this book.

Congratulations and all the best to you & your baby on your journey ahead.

Feel free to replace the words "Angels / Archangels" with words like "God / Deity / Source / Universe" – whatever you believe in, because that is what matters.

It would be great if you can take a minute to signup with us here - http://eepurl.com/btHI9v - to receive amazing free content like Angel prayers, quotations, free e-books & more.

Thanks!

How to use this book

This book is designed to be your companion during the 9 months of your pregnancy. Like a loving friend who encourages you to be grateful for the little joys of life, I wish that this book helps bring you closer to your God and your loving Angels.

There is a set of prayers & affirmations for each week of your pregnancy. Read them with all your heart anytime during the day. Add / modify these prayers to suit your needs, make them truly yours. After all, they are yours.

Each set of prayer / affirmation is divided into 4 parts. First we thank for all the blessings we have, then we bless the baby's developments that are happening this week. Next we pray for our body and at last we request Angels to shield and protect us.

I truly hope that you love this book. Thank you.

A small note from the Author:

Dear Reader,

Thank you for purchasing this book.

Congratulations and all the best to you & your baby on your journey ahead.

Feel free to replace the words "Angels / Archangels" with words like "God / Deity / Source / Universe" — whatever you believe in, because that is what matters.

It would be great if you can take a minute to signup with us here - http://eepurl.com/btHI9v - to receive amazing free content like Angel prayers, quotations, free e-books & more.

Thanks!

How to use this book

This book is designed to be your companion during the 9 months of your pregnancy. Like a loving friend who encourages you to be grateful for the little joys of life, I wish that this book helps bring you closer to your God and your loving Angels.

There is a set of prayers & affirmations for each week of your pregnancy. Read them with all your heart anytime during the day. Add / modify these prayers to suit your needs, make them truly yours. After all, they are yours.

Each set of prayer / affirmation is divided into 4 parts. First we thank for all the blessings we have, then we bless the baby's developments that are happening this week. Next we pray for our body and at last we request Angels to shield and protect us.

I truly hope that you love this book. Thank you.

Dedicated to Moms

& the Archangels

Table of Contents:

Prayer for Angelic Protection

My Dearest God, all the Mighty Archangels, all the Spiritual Masters & Holy Saints. My dear Guides and my loving Guardian Angels – please hear me now.

I request you all to surround me with your divine love and protection today. Please guide me at every moment of my life encouraging me to be the best I can be.

Dear Archangels, please wrap me in your loving wings and pour your divine, radiant white angelic light into my aura. Please cleanse, energize and balance my body at all levels.

I am now fully protected; fully safe and fully loved at all levels of my being. Thank you.

To pray

is to let go

& let God take over.

-Philippians 4:6-7

Pre-conception & Week 1

My dear God and my loving Angels, my partner and I are ready to welcome a lovely, healthy little baby into our lives. As we plan for conception, I am deeply and humbly thankful to you as you bless me, my body and that of my partners. Please prepare our minds, bodies and souls so that we are able to welcome a beautiful soul onto this planet, into our hearts and into our home.

Dear God may we both be fertile grounds for the baby to come so that the new soul can get all the love, all the nourishment, support and care it needs to be born and raised to lead a happy, healthy and a loving life.

Archangel Michael, I request you to wrap us in your loving wings, look after us and protect us throughout this week.

Thank you.

A baby is a bit of stardust

blown from the hands of God

-Barretto

Pregnancy Week: 2

Dear God and my loving Angels, my partner and I are ready and looking forward to welcome a new baby into our lives. We both humbly request you to make us able in all ways to be the best parents we can ever be.

Dear God, may my body be physically, mentally and emotionally fit to nourish my child and raise a happy and healthy baby.

My dearest little child in heaven, please give us the honor to be your parents. Please be our little miracle. Mom and Dad are waiting for you. We love you.

Archangel Michael, I request you to shield us in your white shield of protection and be with us at all times.

Thank you and in full faith.

Making the decision to have a child

– It's momentous. It is to decide forever

to have your heart go outside your body.

–Elizabeth Stone

Pregnancy Week: 3

Dear God and my dear Angels, as my partner and I heartfully try to conceive a child, we humbly pray that you to bless us with an adorable little miracle.

Dear God please bless and strengthen the sperm so that they are healthy and are able to complete their journey to my egg. Please bless and protect my egg so that it can fully lovingly accept the best sperm and fertilize perfectly. Thank you and in full faith.

Archangel Michael, I pray that you help us this week and always be by our side.

Thank you.

Therefore I tell you,

whatever you ask for in prayer,

believe that you have received it,

and it will be yours.

- Mark11:24

Pregnancy Week: 4

Dear God and my dear Angels, please help us in conception. Please bless our bodies, minds and souls as we try to bring a new life on this planet.

We humbly and heartfully pray that the initial conception has been complete in the most perfect way. I pray that my egg has safely settled in my Uterus.

Dear God, please bless and guide my fertilized egg on its journey ahead. Please bless my Uterus as it becomes a safe haven for our baby to grow in. Thank you and in full faith.

Dear Archangel Michael, please surround us with your love and strength throughout this week and protect us.

Thank you.

We made a wish and

you came true.

- Author Unknown

Pregnancy Week: 5

Dear God and my loving Angels, thank you! Thank you for answering our prayers and blessing us with a beautiful soul. We fully open our hearts and our love to this tiny new being and promise to be the best parents we can ever be.

Dear God, as my baby starts to grow this week, please bless his/her Neural tube formation and the little Heart. Let them develop at their best – fully healthy and fully functional at the perfect time.

Please guide me towards eating healthy food and living a healthy lifestyle so that I am fully able to nourish my body and that of my baby's.

Archangel Michael, I request you to shield my baby & me in your white shield of protection and be with us at all times.

Thank you and in full faith.

The Butterflies he used to give me

have turned into little feet.

– Author Unknown

Pregnancy Week: 6

Dear God and my loving Angels, thank you for being with us and protecting us. As we move into the 6th week of my pregnancy; we humbly pray that you look after the growth of my baby's Brain and Nervous systems. Please bless my child so that he/she is growing in perfect harmony and balance.

Dear God, please bless my body so that it can accommodate the changes caused by pregnancy in a perfect way for my highest good.

Please bless both my baby and I in your shield of protection and love. Thank you.

A baby fills a place in your heart

that you never knew was empty.

– Author Unknown

Pregnancy Week: 7

My dear God and my loving Angels, my baby is growing rapidly now. Though I can't see it yet, I thank you from the bottom of my heart for this little bundle of joy.

As my baby's organs and features continue to form, we pray that you foresee my baby's development with love and grace. Please let everything be in perfect harmony, in utmost perfection and let my baby be healthy and perfectly divine.

Dear God, please protect and look after me and my body so that I am protected and safe throughout my pregnancy. Thank you.

Archangel Michael, I request you to wrap us in your loving wings and protect us throughout this week.

Thank you.

The way we talk to our children

becomes their inner voice.

– Peggy O Mara

Pregnancy Week: 8

Dear God and my dearest Angels, it's already the 8th week! I pray that you bless, guide and support all the people who will be involved with the well-being of my child – especially the doctors, nurses, mid-wives and all the care givers.

Please guide them to give us expert support, care and love, both physically and emotionally. Please guide them to support my baby and me in the best possible way with the best available resources. I also pray that all the machinery and instruments that they use also function perfectly.

Finally, my dearest God, please bless my child and me throughout this week.

Dear Archangel Michael, please surround us with your love and strength throughout this week and protect us.

Thank you.

A woman is the full circle.

Within her is the power to create,

nurture and transform.

– Diane Mariechild

Pregnancy Week: 9

Dear God and my dearest Angels, as I enter the 9th week of my pregnancy, we humbly pray that you bless our little baby. Please look after all the growth and development.

As my baby's Digestive and Reproductive systems form and grow this week, we pray that they are in the perfect condition and in utmost grace.

Archangel Michael, please protect me and my baby in your shield of protection and wrap is in your loving wings. Dear God, we pray that my baby is safe and protected at all times.

Archangel Michael, I request you to shield my baby & me in your white shield of protection and be with us at all times.

Thank you and in full faith.

You are my Sun, Moon

and all of my Stars.

–E. E. Cunnings

Pregnancy Week: 10

Dearest God and my loving Angels, I am thankful and grateful that this week my baby has successfully developed all the vital organs and that all of them are functioning perfectly.

My partner and I are grateful for this little miracle, for this little bundle of joy. We pray that our baby be safe, healthy, perfectly nourished, protected and loved at all times throughout my pregnancy.

Dear God and my Archangels, please surround us in your loving wings and guide us perfectly throughout my pregnancy and after.

Dear Archangel Michael, please protect, guide and shield us throughout this week.

Thank you.

Children are not a distraction from more important work. They are The Most important work.

– C. S. Lewis

Pregnancy Week: 11

Dear God and my loving Angels, I thank you from the bottom of my heart for my beautiful baby. This week please bless both of us as my baby grows rapidly.

May my child perfectly receive all the love, nutrients and oxygen it needs to grow into a healthy & happy baby.

Dear God, please guide and help me with my weight gain. Please guide me towards the perfect food to be consumed in the right quantities that will keep my baby and me healthy.

Archangel Raphael, this week please protect, nourish and heal my baby so that it is safe, loved and protected at all times.

Thank you.

We didn't give you the gift of life.

Life gave us the gift of you.

– Author Unknown

Pregnancy Week: 12

Dear God and my lovely Angels, as I complete my first trimester, my partner and I want to thank you from the bottom of our hearts. We are truly blessed to have a baby into our lives. We promise to be the best parents we can ever be and will love this child fully and unconditionally.

Dear God, this week please bless my baby as its brain continues to grow and the vocal chords are formed. Please bless my baby's newly functioning kidneys as they start filtering to keep me baby healthy.

Please bless my body – physically, emotionally and spiritually and protect me.

Dear Archangel Michael & dear Archangel Raphael, please look after me and my baby this week.

Thank you.

So many of my smiles

begin with you.

– Author Unknown

Pregnancy Week: 13

Dear God and my loving Angels, this week please bless my Placenta as it nourishes my baby. Please also guide me towards the right diet and the right intake of vitamins and supplements that are necessary for my baby's perfect growth and over all well being.

Dear God, please give me the strength, courage, love and compassion to bring this lovely soul onto earth and care for it in the best way I can.

Please bless and look after all my baby's growth and development this week with love.

Archangel Michael, I request you to wrap us in your loving wings and protect us throughout this week.

Thank you.

A baby is the greatest of gifts

that life can bring.

– Author Unknown

Pregnancy Week: 14

Dear God and my Angels, as I enter the 14th week of my pregnancy; I pray that you look after my baby's overall growth and development. Please bless my baby's Thyroid gland and let it function in the utmost perfect state.

Please bless my body this week. Guide me towards eating healthy, getting enough exercise, inhaling fresh oxygen and consuming all the vital nutrients to keep my body healthy and my baby nourished.

Dear Archangel Michael, this week I pray that you always be by our side and protect my baby at all times.

Thank you and in full faith.

Dear God in your strong hands,

I place our lives today.

Choosing to depend on you,

to light and guide our way.

– A prayer

Pregnancy Week: 15

My dear God and my dear Angels, I thank you from the bottom of my heart for continually being with us and caring for us.

This week as my baby's skeletal system and muscle development continues to happen, I pray that you look after the growth and ensure that my baby develops perfectly.

Dear God, I request you to bless my body as it changes to accommodate the new baby. Please guide me so that I can care for my body in the best possible way. Thank you.

Dear Archangels, please surround me and my baby in your loving wings and protect us.

Thank you.

You never understand life

until it grows inside of you.

– Sandra C. Kasis

Pregnancy Week: 16

Dear God and my Angels, this week I request you to bless and guide my care givers so that they are at their best while caring for my baby. Please bless all the machinery and instruments they use, so that they function perfectly at all times.

Dear God, please let my baby's growth and development happen in the most perfect way possible. Let my baby feel safe, loved and protected.

Dear Archangel Michael, this week I pray for your support, love and your shield of protection around my baby as it continues to happily grow inside me.

Thank you.

May God help me to keep you safe

And always keep you strong, I pray

I love you right before I planned you

And I love you more now that I have you.

– Danielle Bramlett

Pregnancy Week: 17

Dear God and my loving Angels, as we move to the 17th week of my pregnancy, I want to humbly thank you for being with us all along. Thank you for my little baby, the love of my life.

I pray that my baby always receives the perfect amount of oxygen, nourishment, care and love for him/her to grow fully and perfectly.

Dear God, I request you to bless and support my body as it changes and accommodates my growing child. This week, please bless my breasts as they start to prepare milk for my baby.

Archangel Raphael, I request you to bless, heal and support my body and that of my baby's at all times.

Thank you.

Though I only saw you
as an image on a screen
I still love you,
with every inch of my being.

- Katie C

Pregnancy Week: 18

Dear God and my loving Angels, this week as my baby's eyes, ears and bones continue to grow and function, I request you to look after their growth so that they fully grow and function properly.

Dear God, my partner and I humbly thank you for choosing us as the parents of this beautiful soul. Please help and guide us to be the best of parents and give our baby all the love and support it needs throughout.

As my body is growing, dear God please look after me. Please guide me to all that I need to know and do to stay healthy, happy and strong.

Dear Archangel Michael, please surround us with your love and strength throughout this week and protect us.

Thank you.

I look forward to your birth,

when I can kiss your skin,

but for now I will just smile,

As I feel you play within.

– Author Unknown

Pregnancy Week: 19

Dearest God and my loving Angels, this week as my baby's skin is developing I pray that you bless the development process.

My partner and I are excited, happy and thankful for we can feel the first movements of our child. These loving moments are joyous and out-of-the world. At the same time they remind me of this divine miracle growing inside me.

Dear God, please bless and guide me so that I can lovingly care for my baby in the best possible way.

Dear Archangel Michael, I request your cloak of love and protection for me and my baby throughout this week.

Thank you.

As mother with child our journey's begun,

My heart's yours forever, little one.

I loved you from the very start.

You stole my breath, embraced my heart.

– Author Unknown

Pregnancy Week: 20

My dear God and my loving Angels, as we enter into my 20th week of pregnancy, I deeply and humbly thank you for this little miracle growing inside me. Thank you for this little bundle of joy.

Dear Angels, as my baby continues to grow and develop, please look after all the stages of its development. Let my baby receive – in the best possible way – all the love, nourishment, vital nutrients, oxygen and everything else required for its perfect growth.

Dear God, please bless and care for my body as it changes and adjusts to accommodate my growing baby. Please guide me to the best food, to the best exercises, the best care givers and to the best knowledge sources I need to support my baby in the perfect way possible.

Dear Archangel Michael, please protect and shield us throughout this week.

Thank you.

A grand adventure

is about to begin.

– Winnie the Pooh

Pregnancy Week: 21

Dear God and my dear Angels, thank you for constantly being with me and my baby for the last 20 weeks. As my baby is 21 weeks old now, I pray that you look after its development and growth.

Dear God, please bless my baby's bone marrow as they start producing blood cells this week. Please bless and nourish my placenta as it is the main source of nourishment for my baby.

Dear God and my Angels, I pray that you guide me to eat healthy, take care of my body both physically, mentally and emotionally so that I can lovingly support my child.

Dear Archangel Michael, I request you to lovingly cloak us with your brilliant white shield of light giving us the utmost protection throughout this week.

Thank you.

Children reinvent your world for you.

- Susan Saradon

Pregnancy Week: 22

Dear God almighty and my dearest Angels, I love you. Thank you for blessing us with this beautiful baby.

This week as my baby's senses begin to grow, I pray that you look after and guide their development in a perfect way. Dear God please also bless the development and functioning of my baby's other vital systems.

This week as my body prepares for the upcoming rapid growth of my baby, I request your presence and blessings with me at all times.

Dear God, please guide me towards the best care providers for my baby both during pregnancy and post birth.

Dear Archangel Michael, I pray for your loving golden white shield of protection with me and my baby.

Thank you.

The moment a child is born,

a mother also is born.

She never existed before.

-Osho

Pregnancy Week: 23

My dear God and my loving Angels, we heartfully thank you for this little miracle growing inside me.

Each of my baby's movements brings me joy and hope. I am deeply thankful and grateful for being able to experience pregnancy and motherhood.

Dear God as my baby continues to grow; I pray that you lovingly look after its development. As my own body continues to grow and accommodate my baby, I pray that you guide me to the best way I can care for my body. Dear God, please help me maintain my calm, balance, good health, high spirits and optimism throughout my pregnancy and after.

Archangel Michael, thank you for being with us. Please wrap us in your loving wings and protect us at all times.

Thank you.

Giving birth is an ecstatic jubilant adventure not available to males. It is a woman's crowning creative experience of a lifetime.

– John Stevenson

Pregnancy Week: 24

Dear God and my dearest Angels, thank you for your blessings and love.

This week I pray that you look after my baby's lungs and respiratory systems as they prepare for life outside my womb. Dear God, please bless and look after my baby's movements and overall developments.

Please guide me towards maintaining the best diet, the best daily routine and the best emotional state so that I can fully nurture and support my baby.

Archangel Michael, please be with us this week and shield is in your cloak of protection throughout.

Thank you.

Before you were conceived I wanted you.

Before you were born I loved you.

Before you were here an hour I would die for you.

This is the miracle of Mother's Love.

– Maureen Hawkins

Pregnancy Week: 25

Dear God and my dearest Angels, my baby can hear us now. I feel so wonderful. This makes my bond with my baby even stronger.

Dear God, please bless and guide me to say the right things and provide the right experiences to my baby so that he/she has the perfect values, perfect health and perfect personality when they grow up.

Dear God as my body continues to accommodate my growing child, I pray that you help me consume the right food, find the best care givers, find enough time to rest and everything else I need to fully support myself and my baby in the best way possible.

Archangel Michael, I request you to shield my baby & me in your white shield of protection and be with us at all times.

Thank you and in full faith.

This is the most extraordinary thing

about motherhood – finding a piece of yourself

separate and apart that all the same

you could not live without.

– Jodi Picoult

Pregnancy Week: 26

Dear God and my loving Angels, I thank you for this little miracle growing inside me.

As my little bundle of joy continues to grow each day, I pray that you look after my baby's overall development. Please let him/her receive the right amount of care, love and support it needs to grow perfectly.

Dear God, as my partner and I prepare for life with a baby, we humbly pray that you manifest all the resources, care givers, helpers, knowledge sources & everything else we need so that we can provide the best life for our baby.

We pray that we have the time, the right mindset and the best resources to give our baby the best possible environment to grow.

Archangel Michael, I pray that you help us this week and always be by our side. Thank you.

A mom's hug lasts long after she lets go.

- Author Unknown

Pregnancy Week: 27

Dear God and my dearest Angels, as we enter the 3rd trimester of my pregnancy I thank you from the bottom of my heart. Thank you. Thank you for supporting me and my baby in this journey.

Dear God, this week I humbly pray that you help me be the best mother I can be. As my baby starts to recognize our voices, please guide us to say the right things to our child.

We request your support in providing the best possible environment for my little baby to grown in. Dear God please guide me to learn more about life after delivery and help me find the right support groups, care givers and help.

Archangel Michael, I request you to shield my baby & me in your white shield of protection and be with us at all times.

Thank you and in full faith.

I remember my mother's prayers and they have always followed me. They have clung to me all my life.

- Abraham Lincoln

Pregnancy Week: 28

Dear God and my loving Angels, thank you for supporting my baby and me during the last 27 weeks.

This week as my baby continues to grow, I pray that you look after all my baby's development. Please bless and care for my baby's brain as it continues to grow and expand.

Dear God, please also bless my body as it continues to grow and adjust to support my baby. Please help me receive adequate care, nourishment and rest so that I can provide the best growing environment for my child – both physically and emotionally.

Dear God, please bless us so that we have a perfect pregnancy, child birth and beyond.

Dear Archangel Michael, please protect and shield us throughout this week.

Thank you.

My precious little baby

I have loved you from the start.

You are a tiny miracle

laying closely to my heart.

– Author Unknown

Pregnancy Week: 29

Dear God and my loving Angels, as we move to the 29th week of my pregnancy, I want to humbly thank you for all the support, care and love you have been showering us with.

Dear God, as my baby grows in size and continues to move around, I pray that you look after my baby's movements. Please let everything be in perfect harmony and for my baby's highest good.

Dear God, as my body feeds my growing child, please guide me towards eating a healthy diet and maintaining a healthy lifestyle so that I can provide the best nutrients, care, warmth, oxygen and everything else my child needs to grow perfectly.

Archangel Michael, I request you to wrap us in your loving wings and protect us throughout this week.

Thank you.

When two hearts beat together,

the third one is conceived.

– Whiteracoon

Pregnancy Week: 30

Dear God and my Angels, this week I thank you from the bottom of my heart for blessing us with this beautiful little miracle.

I love my baby and promise to care for my child in the best way I can. Dear God, as my baby practices and prepares for breathing outside of the womb, I pray that you look after and guide my baby's respiratory systems.

As my baby continues to grow in size, please lovingly look after all the stages of my baby's developments.

Dear God, this week please guide me towards eating right and preparing for life with a baby.

Dear Archangel Michael, please surround us with your love and strength throughout this week and protect us.

Thank you.

There is only one pretty child in the world,
and every mother has it.

– Chinese proverb

Pregnancy Week: 31

Dear God and my loving Angels, I love you. Thank you for blessing me with this beautiful baby.

This week I pray that you bless my baby's digestive system and all the other vital organs. Please ensure that all of them are working in perfect condition and in the best coordinated way possible.

Dear God, this week as my breasts have started to prepare for nourishing my baby after birth, I pray that you bless them and look after the changes and developments with love and grace.

Dear God, please always bless us as my partner & I look forward to a fantastic life with a baby.

Archangel Michael and my dear Archangel Gabriel this week I request that you both be with us throughout and wrap us in your loving protective wings.

Thank you.

Being a full-time mother is one of the

highest salaried jobs in my field,

since the payment is pure love.

- Mildred B. Vermont

Pregnancy Week: 32

Dear God and my dearest Angels, as my baby continues to grow and prepare for life outside my womb, we deeply and humbly thank you for this little miracle growing inside me.

Dear God, please always look after and bless my baby. As my body is perfectly and relentlessly supporting this child, I pray that you give me the strength, courage, nourishment and love needed for my body to continue supporting my baby at its best and to heal perfectly after child birth.

Dear Archangel Michael, please look after my child this week and wrap us in your loving and protective shield.

Thank you.

The most important thing she'd learned

over the years was that there was no way to

be a perfect mother and a million ways

to be a good one.

– Jill Churchill

Pregnancy Week: 33

Dear God and my loving Angels, thank you for always being there for us and supporting us during my pregnancy.

As my baby is more aware of its surroundings, can feel my touch and hear my voice, dear God, please guide me so that I can send the best thoughts, say the best words and give him/her the most loving touch I can. Please let me baby feel secure, comfortable, happy and loved.

Dear God and my Angels please also guide me towards the right knowledge sources, the right people, the right care givers who can help me during my upcoming labor in the next few weeks.

Archangel Michael, I request you to guide and protect us this week. Please always be by our side and wrap us in your loving wings.

Thank you.

*You can't imagine your life
with kids until you have them,
then you can't imagine
your life without them.*

- Wise Old Man

Pregnancy Week: 34

Dear God and my loving Angels this week as my body continues to be a loving home for my child, I pray that you bless, support and strengthen me as I support my growing child.

Dear God, please send the perfect help, the perfect support groups and care givers to me so that I receive the right amount of nutrition, exercise and rest that I need.

Dear God, as my baby continues to grow this week, I request you to lovingly look after all the stages of his/her development and let everything be in perfect harmony for the highest good.

My dear Archangel Michael, please wrap us in your white shield of protection this week.

Thank you.

A baby is a blessing.
A gift from heaven above,
a precious little angel to
cherish and to love.

– Author Unknown

Pregnancy Week: 35

Dear God and my loving Angels, as my baby is happily growing and preparing for life after birth, I am thankful and grateful for this little miracle growing inside me.

Dear God, please look after all the stages of my baby's growth and development and let everything be in perfect grace and for the highest good.

Dearest God, I humbly thank you for the amazing and loving bond that my baby and I share. Please help and guide me in giving the best experiences to my child now that will help his/her overall development.

Archangel Michael and Archangel Jophiel, I request you to surround us with your loving energies this week and protect us.

Thank you.

No language can express the power

and beauty and heroism of

a mother's love.

– Edwin H. Chapin

Pregnancy Week: 36

Dear God and my loving Angels, as we enter the 36th week of my pregnancy, I request you to help me start preparing for child birth – both physically and mentally. Please help me gather enough knowledge that will make this process easier.

Please bless my care-givers as they now start to closely monitor my child's development. Dear God, please look after my baby as we approach the last few weeks of my pregnancy and please let everything happen for our highest good.

Dear God, please help my body get the right amount of nourishment, rest and love so that I can give the same to my child.

All the Archangels and Angels, please hear me now. I request you all to be with us throughout this week. Please wrap us in your loving wings and pray for my baby's well being. Please surround us and give us the utmost protection.

Thank you.

I hold my whole world in my arms,

every time I hold my baby.

- Bonnie Ann

Pregnancy Week: 37

Dear God and my loving Angels, thank you for being with us all along, loving us and blessing us throughout my pregnancy.

Dear God, as my baby continues to grow and is aware of its surroundings, please guide me to provide him/her with the most perfect experiences to help in its overall development.

As my body starts to prepare for child birth, dear God; please lovingly look after all the developments and changes taking place in my body. Please give me the courage, strength, love and support I need to fully experience a perfect child birth.

All the Archangels and Angels, please hear me now. I request you all to be with us throughout this week. Please wrap us in your loving wings and pray for my baby's well being.

Thank you.

The only thing worth stealing

is a kiss from a sleeping child.

- Sonia

Pregnancy Week: 38

Dear God and my loving Angels, please bless my baby this week. As my baby grows and all his/her vital organs are now functioning, I pray that you look after each of them in turn with your love and grace.

Please let all of my baby's internal systems be perfectly developed and perfectly functioning. Dear God, as my baby prepares for its journey into the outside world, I pray that you look after my baby and me.

Please give my body enough strength and rest so that I can be fit and fully prepared for my journey ahead. Dear God, please also help me prepare a safe haven for my baby to live in after birth.

All the Archangels and Angels, please hear me now. I request you all to be with us throughout this week. Please wrap us in your loving wings and pray for my baby's well being.

Thank you.

Labor is the only blind date

where you know you will meet

the love of your life.

– Author Unknown

Pregnancy Week: 39

Dear God and my loving Angels, we have almost made it! As I enter into the 39th week of my pregnancy I thank you for being with us all the way.

Dear God, please give my mind, body and spirit the strength and courage I need to deliver a healthy and happy baby into this world. Dear God, please continue to look after and care for my baby fully in the best way possible.

Dear God, please let all the resources, support and love I need during child birth be made available to me and my child at the right time.

All the Archangels and Angels, please hear me now. I request you all to be with us throughout this week. Please wrap us in your loving wings and pray for my baby's well being.

Thank you.

We're growing together.

We are seeing the world like its new.

I will open my heart and love

will rain down all over you.

You'll giggle

and I'll do it all over again.

And we will walk hand in hand

until you let go.

I might have made you,

but You made me a Mother.

– Author Unknown

Pregnancy Week: 40

Dear God and my dear Angels, as my baby and I enter the final week(s) of our pregnancy I thank you for choosing us to the parents of this lovely child.

This week as we wait for my contractions and labor to start, I request that you fully bless and guide all the care-givers that are involved during my child birth. By your grace, may they know the right procedures to follow and take the perfect steps & care to be given to both of us.

Dear God, as we await the birth of my child, please bless and strengthen my body as it is about to experience the most amazing miracle – that of life itself.

Dear God, Dear Archangels, My Guides and My Guardian Angels, I request you all to be with my baby and me throughout the child birth and beyond. Please surround us with your loving energies and give us the utmost protection.

Thank you.

From the Author:

Liked the book? I hope so!

Hi there! I wish that you have found this book helpful in your journey.

If this book has helped you even in the tiniest bit and touched you, please take a minute and rate this on Amazon and leave me a comment. I love hearing your stories and your journeys with this book.

P.S: Please sign up http://eepurl.com/btHI9v to get free Angel prayers, quotations and updates. I won't spam. Promise.

About the Author

Hi! I am Jayasri Nagrale. I am a 30 year young, fun loving, crazy crafter, a student of spirituality & self discovery, a techie and an entrepreneur. I am happily married to my hubby Kranthi.

My spiritual journey started 5 years ago and I am still constantly learning. To be honest, the true authors of this book are Archangel Gabriel and Archangel Uriel.

Bringing this book to the world, to the hands of expectant mothers as a way for them to connect with God and their child – was Archangel Gabriel's idea which she planted in my mind. Archangel Uriel and I then wrote out this whole book – in a week's time!

I am honored to have been chosen to bring this book to you. I hope this book has touched you and helped you in your journey. Thank you.

Thank you

God bless you both.